Tea Cleanse

The Ultimate Beginner's Guide & Action Plan to Tea Cleansing Diet for Weight Loss –

A Natural Solution to Detox & Boost Your Body's Metabolism

By *Jennifer Louissa*

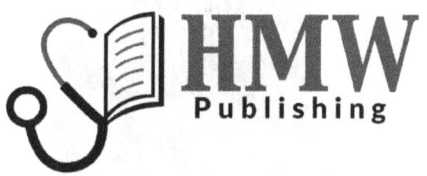

For more great books visit:

HMWPublishing.com

Get another book for Free

I want to thank you for purchasing this book and offer you another book (just as long and valuable as this book), "Health & Fitness Mistakes You Don't Know You're Making", completely free.

Visit the link below to signup and receive it:

www.hmwpublishing.com/gift

In this book, I will break down the most common health & fitness mistakes, you are probably committing right now, and I will reveal how you can easily get in the best shape of your life!

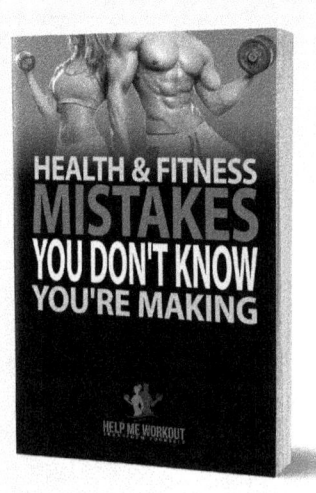

In addition to this valuable gift, you will also have an opportunity to get our new books for free, enter giveaways, and receive other valuable emails from me. Again, visit the link to sign up:

www.hmwpublishing.com/gift

Table of Contents

Book Description 1

Introduction 3

Chapter 1: What are Toxins? 6

    The Different Sources of Toxins 8

    How do Toxins Affect You? 12

Chapter 2: Tea Cleansing in a Nutshell 13

    True Tea for Cleansing? 14

    Builds Your Immune System 16

    Curbs Your Appetite 17

    Helps the Body in Digestion 18

    What Happens Inside Your Body During Cleansing 19

    Important Suggestions Before Starting Tea Cleansing 20

Chapter 3: The Truth About Tea Bags 23

Chapter 4: Best Type of Teas for Cleansing .. 29

Chapter 5: The Benefits of Tea Cleansing 33

    Green Tea: 34

    Black Tea: 34

    Darjeeling Tea: 35

    Blooming Tea: 35

    White Tea: 36

Chapter 6: Proper Tea Brewing 38

    Water 38

Type of Teapots 39
　　Steep Times and Temperature 40
　　Guidelines... 41

Chapter 7: Grading Your Tea Leaves............ 45

Chapter 8: How Do You Choose the Proper Tea for Detoxing 50

　　Full or Broken Leaf Tea? 50
　　What are the Tea Benefits You are After?............ 51

Chapter 9: Cleansing Plan 59

Chapter 10: Reminders and Take-Aways 64

Conclusion 70

Final Words 72

About the Co-Author 73

Book Description

There have been a lot of trips to the gym and never have they ended up in your daily life routine. The gym is good until your school starts again or your boss starts giving you more work, and you realize there is no time for it in your tight routine, and you feel the unnecessary fat under your touch.

The diet plans are stuck in your fridge and trying them has been hard. Eating vegetables and fruits are fun until you feel the lethargy and weakness kick in. It isn't too late when you feel the mood swings coming right at you, and a little too soon, you find yourself eating the greasy food from the nearest junk food place. Reading this, you will know an easy way to lose weight and flush out the toxins.

There is nothing saddening than feeling helpless and not being able to do anything about it. This book will take you step by step and enlighten you about an amazing way to lose weight, and you will be more than happy to use it.

In this book, you will be told about:

- What are toxins and how they are harmful to your body

- What problems you face while losing weight.

- If the toxins stay in your body, how they harm you.

- Cleansing tea is a very simple way to lose weight and fasten your metabolism.

INTRODUCTION

If there is one thing that we do not know about toxins, it is that having them inside our bodies in a certain amount can make it enough for them to earn the label *harmful*.

True enough there are so many ways that different toxins affect us, but one of the most known effects they have is us getting fat. Many of these toxins enter our system as an ingredient of some unhealthy food that we blatantly choose.

Undoubtedly, most of us already went through the phase where we only choose to blame other people and things. Admit it, many of us think that blaming anything other than yourself makes it more comfortable, but think again. Regardless of who you are accusing, it will still not make your health any better.

So, we move on to your sudden urge to finally put things right and tea cleansing, together with other healthy options, suddenly enter the scene. But what is tea cleansing? Is it a viable option to keep trim or does it only cleanse you from the inside? Let us delve deeper into the facts about tea cleansing; you will soon find out why the old world appreciated it so much. Thanks again for purchasing this book, I hope you reading enjoy it and please do not forget to leave us an honest review ☺!

Also, before you get started, I recommend you **joining our email newsletter** to receive updates on any upcoming new book releases or promotions. You can sign-up for free, and as a bonus, you will receive a free gift. Our "*Health & Fitness Mistakes You Don't Know You're Making*" book! This book has been written to demystify, expose the top do's and don'ts and to finally equip you with the information you need to get in the best shape of your life. Due to the overwhelming amount of mis-information and lies told by magazines and self-proclaimed "gurus", it's becoming harder and harder to get reliable information to get in shape. As opposed to having to go through dozens of biased, unreliable and un-trustworthy sources to get your health & fitness information.

Everything you need to help you has been broken down in this book for you to easily follow and to immediately get results to achieve your desired fitness goals in the shortest amount of time.

Once again, to join our free email newsletter and to receive a free copy of this valuable book, please visit the link and signup now: www.hmwpublishing.com/gift

Chapter 1: What are Toxins?

We have been hearing the word *toxins* for such a long time that we have learned to either ignore its true meaning or not even try to find out what it means.

For many, toxins are the things that our body naturally excrete as a part of cleansing and protecting itself. That can be quite right, but that does not precisely answer the what part.

Toxins are harmful agents that can be environmental, biological, and even autogenous. Meaning they from the environment (air, water, the food we eat, and also the chemicals we use in our daily lives) or from the byproducts of our bodies. These things do not cause anything else but harm. In short, they are poison to us. As for autogenous toxins, these are the toxins that we are born with that stems from the generations of toxins that our family is exposed to.

It is also good for you to know that toxins do not only poison your body, they also poison your mind. How so? They creep into your system gently; you will not even feel it until it is already too late. First, they affect your body slowly, hindering it from functioning well. This effect alone can already lead to stress, what with our body trying to find a way to operate as it should, add to that your frustration that lately, you keep on feeling that something is off.

Stress does not only impede you from doing your daily work and from your body to function regularly, but it also ruins your usual pattern, and if left unattended, can lead to burn out. Burn out will not kill you. What will kill you are the complications that it exposes you to. You see, when a person is burned out, his or her immune system goes down and exposes you to a high risk of contracting diseases. That disease you are exposed to will eventually kill you. I'm quite sure nobody wants that to happen to them.

These poisons also have different forms and sources, roughly reaching up to 600 variations, give or take a few. With a list of poisons such as this you can, pretty much, say that almost everything around you contains toxins. So, what does eating have to do with them?

Watching our food intake helps us reduce the toxins that enter or get produced in our bodies. Let me be clear though, watching what we eat does not help us too much with expelling the poisons from our system. The only way for us to discharge these harmful things is by urinating and defecating. As for the belief that sweat helps out in removing them, not really. You can run all day or find a way to sweat excessively. Yes, you will slim down, but the toxins will still be there.

THE DIFFERENT SOURCES OF TOXINS

Air - Toxins from air enter through our skin and lungs.

- Any burning organic compound* is already a toxin because it produces tar that travels through the airway and eventually damages the lungs. A good example is a tar from smoking or second-hand smoking, joystick smoke as a relaxant for massages, yoga sessions, and even tai chi classes.

- Ammonia that can be found in animal urine that has

been standing for days or cigarettes.

- Chemical cleaning products especially those with strong fumes like bleach or muriatic acid.

- Chemical spray such as air fresheners.

- Fumes from fireworks, petrochemical-based products, nail lacquers, hair spray, airplane cabin air, traffic fumes, printer inks, and more.

*organic compound – any solid, liquid, or gaseous compound that contains carbon in its molecules.

Water (not ingested) - Toxins from water enter through our eyes, skin, and air.

- Chlorine, chloroform, hydrogen sulfide, and trichloroethylene that can be absorbed while bathing, especially with hot showers that strip off our body's natural oils and exposes our pores.

- Chloramines, trichloramine, trihalomethanes, and other ammonium compounds (urine, lotion, oil from the skin, flakes from dry skin) that can be absorbed when bathing in ponds, lakes, rivers, and the sea.

Water (ingested)

- Fluoride, chlorine, cadmium from tap water, mineral water, and well water.

- Food

- Including beverages made from powdered juice, coffee, tea, or fruits and vegetables sprayed with chemicals by the growers.

- Additives, food colouring, monosodium glutamate (MSG), preservatives, artificial flavouring, artificial sweeteners and more that can be found on your regular store-bought food.

Chemicals

- Medicines such as antibiotics.

- Vaccines containing mercury or thimerosal (organic

mercury).

- Tattoo ink contains mercury.

- Amalgam fillings containing mercury.

- Shampoo, conditioner, makeup, lotion, mouthwash containing preservatives like paraben, propylparaben, ethylparaben, methylparaben that can trigger your cancer cells. Sulfates, the preservation and foaming agents that cause allergy-like symptoms such as difficulty in breathing or hives. PEG or polyethylene glycol, a thickener, softener, or moisture carrier that reduces the natural moisture of your skin leaving you more exposed to bacteria.

PEG or polyethylene glycol, when indicated on the label for ingredients, is usually followed by a bunch of numbers like PEG-40 or PEG-150. The higher the number that follows the acronym PEG, the safer it is, because the lower number means it is a lot easier for your skin to absorb it.

Good to know: *The human body is exposed to about 200* *types of organic chemicals daily due to the intake of food and its additives, the use of cleaning products, toiletries, and even makeup.*

How do Toxins Affect You?

The truth is that there are many products and things we use in our everyday lives that contain chemicals. These chemicals are all potentially toxic, and once they reach a certain level, that is when they can affect you. How so? Depends on the dosage or the amounts of it that we have in our body. Add to that the fact that we either choose to ignore or do not take caution to their ultimate effects because, well, we do not see them.

We, humans, are used to recognizing harm only when we can see it large and looming right in front of our eyes. Until then, everything seems to go swimmingly for us even if the truth says otherwise.

Chapter 2: Tea Cleansing in a Nutshell

Tea cleansing, for many, is a method of drinking "*dieting or slimming*" tea, fasting, and avoiding a whole bunch of food groups to get the "*toxins*" out of their system that will hasten their slimming down.

This is not how your tea cleansing will go. In fact, nobody's tea cleansing method should go like that, because it is dangerous for your health. You will be using true teas and **tisanes** or herbal teas instead. You will not be forcing your body to do anything. All that you will be doing is gently introducing healthy things into your body, and encouraging it to cleanse your system for it to function well.

Just to be clear, we are not talking about this dieting or slimming tea. We are talking about the true teas and the herbal ones that indeed give you health benefits.

TRUE TEA FOR CLEANSING?

So, herbal teas are known to be used for tea cleansing; there is no problem with that. But true teas? Is there such thing – cleansing with true teas?

Yes, there is such thing. Trust me. Before I even started with loose leaves (by the way, let me tell you that if you start going for loose leaves, you will not go back), I used to consume true tea in teabags, just because I wanted to. I did not intend to get slimmer; I just want to feel warmer and lessen my coffee consumption. I had this fixation with Earl Grey; it is a kind of black tea.

Two weeks passed, I still drink my Earl Grey a cup or two daily. Then I noticed my metabolism became better, like everyday-bowel-movement kind of better. Some of my clothes that chafed did not chafe anymore. All my clothes are a comfortable fit. I slept better, plus I felt lighter, never bloated. And that was just a two-week consumption of black tea. Imagine doing that using green tea.

Plus, come on, if true tea is not for tea cleansing, then how do you explain the ridiculously long lives of the old Chinese people and other East Asians who did nothing but drink tea? They drink tea in the morning, at noon, in the evening, during and after meals, drink it just for fun, when sick, in birthdays and all the time. Tea is like water for them, and that is saying something because they consume true tea.

First things first, you have to know that we have options for the kind of tea that you want to use. Our tea options are green tea, black tea, white tea, oolong, rooibos, peppermint, Darjeeling, dandelion tea, and other blooming teas.

With all these options, your body goes on a natural detoxification, without you having to force it to go to that mode. It would be a good thing for you to know that forcing your body to go to detox mode is quite dangerous, so doing that is out of the question.

Your detoxification will take place naturally. It will not impede you from your daily activities; you do not need to fast or go hungry altogether. All you need to do is drink your tea daily, watch your food portioning, throw in a bit of exercise, and all is well. In fact, you can even drink the tea just because you want to drink it. Just enjoy it and while your body is gradually healing and protecting itself.

You do not need to wait for a whole day off from work so that you can drink your tea and worry about a rumbling stomach and annoying toilet sessions for the rest of the day. That is not going to happen with these classic tea options.

BUILDS YOUR IMMUNE SYSTEM

You will find that regardless of the type or flavour of the tea you use for cleansing, they are all good for your immune system because they can strengthen it.

All of the classic herbal teas contain an antioxidant that is highly beneficial to your body, especially the black, white, and green tea.

CURBS YOUR APPETITE

Yes, teas can curb your appetite. While there is some tea that specializes in this function naturally, it would be good for you to know that teas, in general, are useful in curbing your appetite. It makes you feel fuller longer than before you drank your tea. You know why?

Catechins! With lots of antioxidants that you can find in all of these natural teas, surely catechin is one of the antioxidants it contains. It encourages your body to use up your extra fat storage, so, it is all good for you.

However, another good thing that catechins do is balancing your blood sugar. It does so by slowing down the elevation of your blood sugar levels. How?

You see, sugar to travel in our system, needs to be bound to a blood cell. Once it goes in our system and gets to a certain high level, the insulin in our pancreas gets triggered. Insulin will then, start using those sugar in our blood and converts them into energy for us to use or, if we have enough energy, stores them so that insulin can easily turn them for future use once our energy runs out.

That whole process is being slowed down by catechins, in turn, you get blood (without sugar) that circulates in your system while sugar is being held under control by catechins. With tea drinking, your threshold for energy to be used becomes increased, encouraging your body to use its fat reserves. Then it slows down the binding of sugar to your blood, efficiently keeping your blood sugar and insulin levels in balance. If your blood sugar is balanced, your body will not ask your brain to signal you for food supply.

HELPS THE BODY IN DIGESTION

Teas help your body because they have these anti-inflammatory properties that protect your digestive system from being upset. Drinking it hot also aids in cleaning your gut.

If you put an oily food inside the fridge and you see the oil start to solidify, that is pretty much what happens inside your gut if you love eating greasy foods and then drinking something cold afterward. So, regular drinking of hot tea gradually cleanses your stomach of this muck, resulting in smoother digestion. Plus, if you drink hot tea after a meal, it helps with the absorption a lot faster.

What Happens Inside Your Body During Cleansing

Well, apart from better digestion or curbing your hunger, drinking tea encourages sweating. And no, you are not sweating because your body is getting rid of the toxins in it.

You are sweating because your body is trying to cool down, to keep everything inside your body working flawlessly. If you drink something cold, your body will try to cope by making more heat; however, if you drink something hot or warm, your body will deal with it by **regulating** the temperature inside it that often results to you feeling colder. Such bonus.

And so, drinking hot tea in summer is not such a bad idea. This explains why tea drinkers often feel refreshed after a cup of hot tea, as opposed to drinking something cold that makes them more thirsty.

Tea also burns calories with the help of caffeine. Caffeine encourages your body to use more energy resulting in more calories being consumed in the process.

IMPORTANT SUGGESTIONS BEFORE STARTING TEA CLEANSING

As opposed to the popular method people use when tea cleansing such as fasting, our tea cleansing method focuses on the natural methods. It just makes sense because we will be using what we call true teas or that tea that come from the plant *Camellia Sinensis* and other herbs that produce, not dieting or slimming teas that are already processed and added with unknown and weird ingredients.

1. Eat, never starve yourself.

You do not need to avoid a whole food group. All you need is *avoid processed food* as much as possible. This includes junk food, anything with MSG or monosodium glutamate, soda, processed meat.

In cases where you cannot avoid them, make sure you keep to your tea drinking routine to help your body get rid of the toxins it got from such foods.

Also, never even try to fast. You do not need to fast for the tea to start helping your body with the detoxification and other processes. Plus, going hungry will just ruin your metabolism yet, again.

2. Do not drink your tea cold.

Unless you just want to drink it without being concerned about the benefits that hot tea can give you. You see, tea that is left too long until it has gone cold does not taste as good anymore. Plus, hot water just brings out the best in tea such as your antioxidants.

3. Choose your tea well.

Choose which tea is best for you. It can be the flavour or the benefits. The one that you love most works best.

Chapter 3: The Truth About Tea Bags

Ah, one thing that tea purists will insist is that loose leaf teas are better. Then again, tea bags are cheaper, plus it gives you the same good stuff, and flavour, right?

Not exactly. I hate to burst that practicality bubble of yours but there is more to tea bags than just tea, and often, it does not mean good news.

Whenever watching a Japanese or Chinese movie, or any movie that involves the East Asian culture, at one point, you will see them pouring a pot of tea for a guest. So, let me ask you something. Have you ever seen them dipping a tea bag in the teapot for steeping? No, right?

That is because initially, tea is being enjoyed by boiling the leaves - like full, actual plant leaves. Those leaves swell a little, then get soggy and wilted when being boiled. This straightforward and seemingly dull process means a lot when it comes to tea.

Now, imagine suppressing that little leaf-swelling phase of the tea leaves inside a tea bag while boiling them. Ha! It does nothing! – Not really.

You see, tea manufacturers place their premium teas in a can. Inside that can are loose leaves, NOT INDIVIDUALLY-WRAPPED BAGS. And they call it the premium for a reason. Those tea leaves in the can are whole leaves, not broken, not powdered or crushed. These cans mostly go to different tea stores, not in the supermarket.

Now, when you have picked all the whole tea leaves from the bunch, placed them in their beautiful cans, you are left with broken leaves and crushed powdered leaves. Some of those broken leaves go inside beautiful cans as well but are being sold cheaper than the full-leafed ones. Most of these cans go to the supermarket to be sold.

So, with the full leaves tea in their cans, the broken leaves in their cans as well, you are left with crushed minuscule leaves, dust, and powdered tea. They go inside little tea bags that are, then, individually wrapped, placed in boxes, and straight they go to the supermarket. They are the cheapest of the bunch.

Another method for manufacturers to produce mass tea (high volume, low quality) is through the use of a machine that uses the CTC method, or Crush-Torn-Curl, to produce pellets formed out of tea leaves. These pellets are then placed inside the teabags, et voila! You now have your cheap tea.

So, what's the problem with their packaging?

Well, tea leaves have tannins. Tannins give tea the astringent properties and the bitter flavour. Some contain low amounts of it like white tea and green tea.

Now, when full leaf teas are boiled, tannins get released a couple of seconds after. This gives the tea that slight aroma kick and a little bitterness, but that's all good. If your full leaf tea does not give you this little bit of bitterness or astringent feel when boiling it, it might mean it is low quality or old stock. The same story goes for broken tea leaves, except, the tannins create a bit more bitter taste to the tea.

As for the powdered left-over tea leaves, if you accidentally forgot that you are steeping it, left it in there a tad bit longer, once you drink it do not be surprised if you get that medicine-like bitterness from your supposedly lovely cup of tea. Because that is the consequences of crushed tea, it has more tannins than you would want and even if you steep it carefully, you will still get a bitter taste.

Add to that the fact that even if there is a whole bit of tea leaf that got accidentally included in the tea bag, the leaves are still there stuck in that packet. The tea bag will never let them float and get the water they need to expand and bring out the true smell and flavour of the tea.

Then again, if you are not the type who cares so much about the taste of your tea, or you just love its bitter taste, then you would think that it should be no problem at all, right?

Again, not really. This is because apart from more tannins being released from tea bags and less flavour, you also get fewer benefits.

Those antioxidants and catechins I mentioned in the previous chapters? You are likely not going to get them from these tea bags. This is because once a tea leaf has been crushed or broken, the essential oils that it contains that helps create the flavour and scent, are lost. Whatever is left in that tea bag of yours are remnants of the tea leaf's full-flavoured glory.

So, what to do now? What if you still want to save up and you do not want to stock on big canisters of loose leaf teas, or you just want to try a flavour and such?

Well, I suggest that you go for those companies that produce pyramid-shaped tea bags. They are a tad bit expensive than your regular bland-tasting tea bags, but it's going to give you a good taste test for the full-leafed ones in the can.

Pyramid-shaped tea bags have a bigger room that allows the leaves to swim when dipped in boiling water. This enables the leaves to expand and release the flavour. What's more, they also contain full leaves or broken leaves at worst. But that's it, no crushed or powdered leaves.

Chapter 4: Best Type of Teas for Cleansing

1. Green, Black, and White Tea

For the green, black, and white tea, what you have to remember about them is the ingredient call catechin.

Catechins are antioxidants. First, antioxidants. We take Vitamin C for this reason, we need antioxidants, and we have no other choice but to find an external source for this particular component because the body cannot produce it on its own. Antioxidants help strengthen your immunity system, protects you from common illnesses and frightening diseases as well such as cardiovascular diseases and cancer.

That being said, of course, we all want the antioxidant and one type of it is what we call catechins found in black, white, and green tea. So you drink tea like it is a regular, uncomplicated day, and you now have your antioxidant. Easy just like that.

The good thing about catechins is that it does not only keep you safe from a myriad of illnesses and continues to protect you, they are also the one responsible for creating the flavour in your tea and other drinks like wine.

Now, let us focus on the catechins found in tea. What does it do? It helps you slim down by *increasing the allowed amount* of energy that your body can use than its usual amount. This way, all those sitting fats in our bodies, waiting for forever to be used, are *finally* converted into energy and then put to use. This results in weight loss.

2. Oolong Tea

Oolong tea, on the other hand, has so many antioxidants and it mostly works by boosting your metabolism. So, if you have a problem with your daily morning business, might as well choose oolong tea to regulate that before you move on to slimming down.

3. Rooibos Tea

For rooibos tea, well, if you are entirely new to tea drinking or you are a sweet tooth, you will appreciate this tea better than the other ones. You see, rooibos is a tad sweet without you having to add anything to it. You get to enjoy the natural sweetness without worries, plus you also get the benefits of its component, **aspalathin**. Aspalathin helps you curb your stress-induced hunger by reducing your stress hormones. So, no more stress eating.

4. Peppermint Tea

Peppermint tea is obviously peppermint flavoured, so if you are a lover of anything that has to do with this specific flavour, you are always free to choose this tea. The good thing about this is that it suppresses your appetite, no additional ingredients to be added. It is just that, all natural. Also, it is a little sweet, so it is indeed a treat to those who are cutting back on sugar to keep healthy.

5. Dandelion Tea

Dandelion tea is a natural diuretic. Meaning it will encourage your liver to keep processing the water in your body and eliminate it, including toxins. If you suffer from heartburn, then this is an excellent natural treatment for you to keep it at bay. It also helps you balance your blood glucose levels.

Chapter 5: The Benefits of Tea Cleansing

Detoxing has been one of the many fads lately, inspired by celebrities who have so much money, they do not even know which thing they are spending their money on is keeping them trim. They just show you they are trim.

Then again, many studies and research have already exposed the not-so-good side of detoxing. This is where tea cleansing comes in. It is a lot easier approach to keeping healthy and trim than the bothersome detoxing.

So, apart from the fact that tea lowers your risk of stroke, heart disease, reduce your blood pressure, increase your mood and mental performance, what else does it do?

Well, like mentioned earlier, it boosts your energy. In effect, it helps prevent you from gaining extra and unwanted weight.

GREEN TEA:

Usually in packed leaves or powder form. Matcha, a type of green tea, contains five times more L-theanine than the usual green tea.

L-theanine is a component that can be found in teas taken from Camellia Sinensis. It helps give relaxation without making you feel drowsy.

- Antibacterial
- Fights diabetes
- Prevents dementia
- Lowers cholesterol levels
- Fights bad breath
- Helps reduce stress
- Strengthens teeth

BLACK TEA:

The type of tea that contains high levels of anti-oxidants.

(Assam, Earl Grey, Darjeeling, Keemun, Yunan, Ceylon, Bai lin)

- Highly effective in flushing out the toxins in your body
- Has more antioxidants than any other teas, which is vital in preventing cancer

DARJEELING TEA:

Another type of black tea

- Helps calm and soothe your mind
- Has high antioxidant

BLOOMING TEA:

The flashiest of all the teas. Very beautiful to look at, blooms while steeping in water. (Dandelion, Coriander, Cardamom, Cinnamon, Jasmine, Licorice, Ginger, and Sage)

- Helps your metabolism, makes it function smoothly

- Lowers cholesterol
- Balances blood sugar levels
- Gets rid of halitosis or bad breath
- Strengthens and cleans the digestive tract
- Improves immune system
- Helps reduce GERD or acid reflux
- Calms the irritation in your stomach's lining
- Diuretic (

White Tea:

Made from the youngest Camellia Sinensis leaves.

- Contains more antioxidants as compared to Green Tea
- Has anti-aging properties to slow down the process of wrinkling skin
- Protects you from UV rays

- Helps people with diabetes from excessive thirst and increased secretion of insulin

- Helps maintain your reproductive health in good condition

Chapter 6: Proper Tea Brewing

Let us say that you have already chosen your tea, what's next? You are going to make your tea now. Surely you know how to boil water, and you think it is just that easy. Well, it could be, if you do not care about how your tea is going to taste and if your brewing style will bring out the best components in it – that is unless you are a professional tea sommelier.

Water

Best option: Spring or Purified water.

The best water to use for steeping tea is purified or spring water because they do not contain pollutants that can change the taste of the tea. If your water is rich in natural minerals, chances are it will bring out better flavours of your tea.

You may think opting for distilled water is good, but dead water brings out bland or flat tasting tea, nobody likes that.

As for boiled tap water, it is also not a good option for tea brewing. Because it might have already been contaminated by the substances that are flowing in the water pipes and it can positively alter the tea's taste.

Type of Teapots

You know how water can affect the taste of tea? The same can be said for the teapot that you use. So, you do not just go to a tea shop and grab some random teapot to deal with it. If you genuinely want to bring out the best flavours and benefits of your tea, you will have to brew it right. Meaning the water, the duration of brewing, water temperature, and the pot should be the right ones because those things I just mentioned contribute to the result of the tea.

So, for you to have the teapot, you must first have your tea or at least know which tea you are buying the teapot for.

Teas that need high temperatures to bring out the best flavours are best partnered with teapots that are good in retaining heat. On the other hand, teas that need to be brewed at lower temperatures need teapots that will release heat in order not to over brewing them.

Now, there are light teapots, and there are ones that are quite heavy. The ones that are heavy are usually the ones that are good at retaining heat. So you buy them if you choose to have black tea or pu-erh (fermented) tea. On the other hand, tea that is more delicate and can easily get ruined through over brewing, like white or green tea, needs a teapot that can release the heat. This means glass or porcelain teapots is your best option for such tea.

STEEP TIMES AND TEMPERATURE

If there is anything that you need to put in mind when it comes to brewing tea, that would be this:

Each type of tea has a specific temperature level required for you to brew it properly.

The one-size fits all principle do not apply to the water for tea brewing. Following the correct water temperature for each type of tea will help you bring out its best flavour and benefits.

With temperature level, also comes the length of time the tea should be steeped. Again, the one-size fits all principle does not apply here. Before this chapter ends, I will give you a list of the steep times and proper temperature. Then again, once you have tried to follow the correct steep time for your chosen tea and you feel like it is too weak or strong for you, you can always follow your heart to get the right amount of flavour you want. As it is, we will first start walking before we run, or you risk wasting those precious tea leaves.

GUIDELINES

1. Make sure you have your purified water or freshly drawn spring water. Prepare the teapots and the teacups as well.
2. Let the water boil gently in a kettle.
   (Gentle boil means when you look at the water when you think it is already boiling, there is a gentle, yet steady stream of bubbles on the surface. We are not after the angry kind of boiling water where the bubbles start to occupy the whole kettle and starts to look like it is going to come out and chase you anytime soon.)

3. Now, gently pour the hot water into the teapot. Pour some boiling water into each teacup as well. This is to warm the cups so that when you and your friends or family start drinking the tea, you get to enjoy the consistency of flavour because of the cup temperature.
4. Add the tea leaves, making sure you measure it _based on the number of people that will drink the tea_.
5. Let the water cool until it reaches the suggested temperature for the tea and then adds the tea leaves.
6. Let the water cool until it reaches the suggested temperature for the tea and then add the tea leaves.
7. Now, remember your steeping time. It depends on which tea leaves you are using. Steep the tea based on the correct steeping time, wait, and time it. You should be as precise as you can.
8. Once the tea has steeped correctly, you can strain or transfer it to another serving teapot or pour it directly into the teacups.

Tea	Measurement	Steep Time	Temperature	Teapot
Black Tea				
Full Leaf	1-2 teaspoons	2-3 minutes	203°F	Porcelain
Broken Leaf	1-2 teaspoons	3-5 minutes	203°F	Porcelain
Green Tea				
Chinese	2 teaspoons	2-3 minutes	176° - 185°F	Glass/Porcelain
Japanese	1-2 teaspoons	3-5 minutes	203°F	Glass/Earthenware

Oolong Tea Light (Green) Heavy (Dark)	2-3 teaspoons 3-2 teaspoons	2-3 minutes 3-5 minutes	185° - 203°F 203°F	Porcelain/ Yixing Porcelain
Pu-Erh Tea	1-2 teaspoons	3 minutes	212°F	Yixing
Tisanes (Herbal Tea)	1-2 teaspoons	3 minutes	212°F	Glass/ Porcelain
White Tea	2-3 teaspoons	3 minutes	176° - 185°F	Glass/ Porcelain

Chapter 7: Grading Your Tea Leaves

How tea leaves graded? We base it on the traditional preparation or processing of tea leaves in China. After all, that is where it all started.

Then again, it would be good for you to know that the Chinese people themselves understand the proper processing of tea leaves by heart, but do not label the process as such. Grading of tea leaves is used in countries such as Sri Lanka or India, anywhere in the world except China.

Now, why is grading important? If you value your health so much and you intend to give your body the best tea that your money can buy, you will have to have an inkling about tea grading. Either that or you just make your way to the store, buy your whole tea leaves, and you're done. That method does not work for everyone, though.

To those who prefer precision and knowing their money's worth. Here are the categories for grading the leaves:

1. Size – Are the tea leaves big or small? Are they full or broken?

    For this category, small, full leaves are preferred because it means younger leaves are used.

2. What kind of tea leaves are used? Is it made of young leaves or mature ones?

    The younger the leaves, the more delicate tea it yields. If you see tips or small whole leaves, that means you might just have the best bunch of leaves from the entire plant. Seeing the tips from a bunch of processed tea indicates sweet notes once it is brewed. The tips have all the nutrients as well.

Full Leaf Teas

OP (Orange Pekoe)	Consists of the top two leaves

FOP (Flowery Orange Pekoe)	Made from the tips and top two leaves
GFOP (Golden Flowery Orange Pekoe)	Has more tips proportion than FOP
TGFOP (Tippy Golden Flowery Orange Pekoe)	Has more tips proportion than GFOP
FTGFOP (Finest Tippy Golden Flowery Orange Pekoe)	High-quality FOP
STGFOP (Special Finest Tippy Golden Flower Orange Pekoe)	Best quality FOP

*If the grade is added with '1' at the end (FOP1 or STGFOP1), it means that it is the finest quality within that grade.

Broken: Means the leaves are broken and will be used for bagged teas.

Orange:	Not about tea flavour. Orange may suggest the association of tea to the House of Orange when it became popular in the west. May also pertains to the colour of the leaf. A high-quality tea leaf turns into a copper colour when fully oxidized.
Pekoe or Orange Pekoe:	Uncertain origin. Used to describe the presence of tips or budding leaf found on the tea plant.
Tips:	Unopened leaves of the plant.
Tippy:	Teas with the presence of tips from younger leaves are

labeled with the term "tippy."

Broken Leaf Teas

BOP (Broken Orange Pekoe)	Consists of broken top two leaves
FBOP (Flowery Broken Orange Pekoe)	Made from the tips and top two broken leaves
GBOP (Golden Broken Orange Pekoe)	Has more tips proportion than FOP, broken
TGBOP (Tippy Golden Broken Orange Pekoe)	Has more tips proportion than GBOP, broken
GFBOP (Golden Flowery Broken Orange Pekoe)	Best quality FBOP

Chapter 8: How Do You Choose the Proper Tea for Detoxing

Now that you know the grading, it is time for you to choose the proper tea for you. So, do you prefer full leaf tea or broken tea?

Full or Broken Leaf Tea?

Choosing full leaf tea will mean you have the more delicate tea, they are expensive and promises the true flavour of that type of tea that you want. However, that would also mean you will have to steep them longer because full leaves take longer to steep. They promise the true flavour of the tea, but it will be subtle. Subtle flavours are good if you love how they hint you with the different notes of the tea leaves. It keeps you wanting for more without overwhelming you with the flavour. If this description sounds useful to you and you are willing to shell out for an excellent tea, then this is the best choice for you.

However, if you are a lover of bold flavours, you might want to go for broken tea leaves. Now, just because the tea leaves are broken, it does not automatically indicate that you got the lowest quality there is. Remember, there are the fanning and the dust in tea bags to claim the "lowest quality" label. As for broken tea leaves, some of them will still contain the tips that make your tea experience sweeter. Also, broken tea leaves steep faster. This is an excellent choice for you if you are not the type who likes to wait a little longer.

What are the Tea Benefits You are After?

Now that we are done with the technicalities, we proceed to the personal part. What are the benefits of the tea you are after? Would you like to get slimmer? Would you want to keep your system clean? Do you have problems with your metabolism and your daily bowel movement? Would you like to avoid cancer and other deadly diseases? Do you want to stay calm or focused?

It depends on what you want and what your body needs. Of course, you should consider what your body needs first, and if you think that it has already improved or have reached the state that you want, you may move on to *what you truly want*.

Below is a list that contains the many benefits of some of the best tea that you can use for tea cleansing. While all the teas promote weight loss, some of them are more effective. Feel free to check the list and get the tea that gives you the most beneficial effects.

TEA	BENEFITS
Black Tea	- reduces the risk for atherosclerosis
- reduces the risks for kidney stones
- prevents osteoporosis
- helps with weight loss
- helps cure intestinal disorders
- helps relieve asthma
- balances the blood pressure
- helps prevent cancer
- helps maintain your oral health
- gets rid of toxins in the body
- gives focus and mental alertness
- helps prevent heart disease
Chamomile (Tisanes)	- gets rid of diarrhea
- helps alleviate anxiety
- helps alleviate mouth swelling

Dandelion (Tisanes)	• helps cure a hangover • has antimicrobial properties • helps alleviate premenstrual symptoms • lowers high cholesterol levels • helps relieve gastrointestinal issues • helps manage diabetes • helps manage hypertension • boosts the function of liver and kidneys
Ginger (Tisanes)	• gets rid of nausea • helps alleviate morning sickness • gets rid of dizziness • helps relieve menstrual pain
Ginseng	• lowers high blood sugar levels • balances the blood pressure • enhances mental function • cures erectile dysfunction

Green Tea	- helps with weight loss
- boosts your metabolism
- reduces high cholesterol levels
- gives focus and mental alertness
- oral leukoplakia
- cervical dysplasia
- balances the blood pressure
- prevents osteoporosis
Oolong Tea	- provides focus and mental alertness
- helps with weight loss
- boosts metabolism
- encourages healthy skin
- helps keep your bones healthy
- helps prevent cancer
- helps relieve stress

Peppermint (Tisanes)	- helps alleviate stomach pain
- gets rid of bloatedness
- helps relieve stress
- strengthens immune system
- helps with weight loss
- helps relieve asthma
- prevents halitosis or bad breath
- relieves muscle pain and fatigue
- helps relieve chest congestion
- helps cure migraine, nausea, and vomiting
Pu-Erh Tea	- gives focus and mental alertness
- prevents atherosclerosis
- helps with weight loss
- helps prevent cancer
- has anti-aging properties
- has anti-radiation properties
- protects your dental health
- protects the lining of stomach

White Tea	- helps with weight loss
	- has antibacterial and antiviral properties
	- helps in managing diabetes
	- helps maintain reproductive health in good condition
	- helps prevent cancer
	- has anti-aging properties
	- reduces risk of cardiovascular disease
	- protects the skin from UV rays

If you do not like tea cleansing with true teas, of course, you are free to choose any from the tisanes. Just do not veer away from your choices between true teas and tisanes. Never opt for commercialized slimming or dieting teas as you are not sure what other chemicals they contain. They are already too processed to claim to be natural.

There are other tisanes or herbal tea that are also good for tea cleansing such as milk thistle tea, cayenne pepper tea, burdock tea, red clover tea, hibiscus tea, garlic tea, cilantro tea, and chicory tea. In fact, there is a whole lot of choices for you out there; they may be true teas, or tisanes (herbal), it merely depends on the benefits that you want.

Chapter 9: Cleansing Plan

Now that we have, pretty much, everything in place, let us now move on to your tea cleansing plan. Again, let me remind you that you should never starve yourself, it's not such a good idea, plus it defeats the purpose of taking in tea that will improve your metabolism.

Remember, having too much of anything is wrong. Having none is just as bad.

However, there are ones that you need to avoid or lessen the consumption of for the cleansing plan to take effect properly. Here they are:

- cigarettes or tobacco
- alcohol
- coffee
- sugar
- honey

- artificial sweeteners

Lessen the consumption of:

- dairy products

You may also have your true teas decaffeinated if you find them a little too bold for you or if it prevents you from having a good night's sleep.

Feel free to enjoy:

- any fresh fruit

- any fresh vegetables

- raw unsalted almonds, walnuts, macadamias, and cashews

- legumes – can be dried or canned, such as kidney beans, chickpeas, lentils

- lean red meat, chicken (without the skin).

- Eggs: preferably organic

- Olive oil (preferably extra virgin), Coconut oil (unprocessed)

- Seeds: raw unsalted sesame, pumpkin, and sunflower seeds

- Water: from one to three liters of water per day

- Fish: fresh, canned in water or olive oil

A few tea cleansing recipes to help you through your day are,

- Green Tea Cleansing Drink

- Cleansing Dandelion Tea

- Fresh Cranberry Juice

- Fruit mix drink

- Strawberry Banana Yogurt Smoothie

- Cherry Chocolate Milk Smoothie

- Blue Rose Cucumber Smoothie

- Kale and Celery Smoothie

Surely, with all the information here, you should be able to start your cleansing tea diet. Make sure you follow them as much as possible. Tea cleansing will help you shed a few pounds, of course, it depends on how religious you will be on sticking to your plans.

Take advantage of the fact that tea stores are available near you. You can, pretty much, find tea anywhere. You can even order them online. If there is anything that you should be doing right now, that would be re-examining yourself and finding out which tea will give you the benefits you need. Start the healthy routine as soon as you can.

Chapter 10: Reminders and Take-aways

Now that we have reached the end of the book, it would be nice to leave you some parting reminders and takeaways, so here goes:

- As for your metabolism, since you are just about to start your tea cleansing, you need not worry about how messed up your metabolism is. You are not the only one who is having a hard time with it. It will soon get sorted out, and once it does, you can start trying other teas to experience their benefits.

- Tea cleansing is also meant to help calm your mind so you can quickly focus on the things that needed your utmost attention. It also naturally enhances your metabolism, regardless of your age. You know it is true how metabolism slows down as we age, and some of us even start thinking as if there is no way they can fix it anymore. In fact, you can adjust the metabolism issue with just warm water every morning, around 30 minutes after you wake up. However, adding tea to it just makes it more fun, flavourful, the effects are even faster, plus you are showered with more benefits than only one. So, why stick to only plain water, right?

- You may also try performing some meditation for 15 minutes every day. The benefits of your tea consumption, such as better focus, will be enhanced by doing the meditation.

- When eating, feel free also to try your best to cut down, if not avoid altogether, the dressings. I understand, they make the salad less bland, but they are not as healthy as they seem.

- Salads contain enzymes that help your digestion. Enzymes work by breaking down molecules, in this case, your fat molecules. That means you are taking in food and drinks that all focus on keeping you healthy and trim. The effects of what you eat complement each other, so do not be surprised if you start seeing the results in a week or two. Trust me;

tea is one of the few things that exist that shows fast results.

- I know I have mentioned this earlier already, but repeating it just for the sake of gently reminding you would not hurt. So, remember to watch the portioning of what you eat. If you love chocolates, eat a portion of it, wait for about 20 minutes, then drink your favourite tea. That way, the tea makes sure that nothing sticks or gets stuck in your digestive tract. The same thing applies to everything else that you like to eat. Portioning and then tea drinking.

- True tea has steeping guides because they are a bit too sensitive, especially if you opt to buy the more exceptional lot. Tisanes have steeping time as well, but really, it depends on how much flavour you want from the herbal tea. They are not as sensitive as true tea.

- Also, never drink tea on an empty stomach. It might prove to be a little too harsh for an empty stomach, even if your tea of choice is meant to protect your stomach's lining. **<u>Always remember: Eat first, wait for 20 minutes, then drink your tea.</u>** You know, that 20-minute rule is not weird. It does not exist for tea only. In fact, that is how it should be even if you are just drinking plain, room temperature water. The 20-minute rule does magic with your metabolism.

- Add lemon to your tea if you think the flavour is a little too bold for you. Lemon will make it taste lighter, with a spike. If you have cinnamon, you can try adding that to your tea instead of lemon. Apart from discovering new flavours by adding them to your tea, you also get the benefits that they offer.

- There are teas that curbs hunger and cravings. So, in case your cravings suddenly attack at an ungodly hour, drink that hunger-curbing tea instead. You will not only prevent yourself from snacking mindlessly in the middle of the night, but you will also have a better sleep.

- Tea cleansing does not only clean your gut and the

rest of your system, but it also gets rid of the negative energy around you. It makes you feel refreshed, and lighter. It naturally enhances your mood and makes you a calmer. If you choose the right kind of tea, it can help you go to sleep, focus, or just calm down. Do not restrict yourself with only a little information. Feel free to read more about teas. It is such a marvel to discover how beneficial these seemingly very simple drinks are.

- If you enjoy your tea in teabags, do not throw the tea bags after one brew. You can still brew them for the second time. However, the tea will be a bit weaker by then. Again, it is your choice if you will drink the tea, or just place the used bag in the freezer. That used tea bag does wonders for puffy eyes and even acne. Now, you see how excellent tea is? It cleans you from the inside out.

- So, you want something sweet that does not taste like tea, but you are not doing anything about it because you know you will soon feel guilty? Fret no more. You may enjoy hot chocolate, from cocoa tablea. It is best experienced when appropriately crushed. And you will not feel guilty because it is, pretty much, as good as the tea. It is also packed with anti-oxidants. Feel free to enjoy it from time to time when you are craving for coffee or something else other than tea.

- If you want to enjoy your tea cold, steep it in hot or warm water first. You may follow the guide for steeping true teas using the recommended temperature of water. Once appropriately steeped, you may transfer it to a glass and let it cool for a bit. Add ice and enjoy.

There are different ways and tastes of every tea, and whatever suits you best is your choice. A person is not restricted to one kind of tea. I only suggest that you address what ails you first because that is the most sensible thing to do. Something that ails you is not something that can afford to wait, or you risk aggravating it. Once you are done with whatever it is that ails you, then you can try the other flavours for fun, for their benefits, or for flavour hunting.

Conclusion

Check your journal and imprint a week where you have a total separation from capacities or occasions that may crash your cleansing diet, for example, weddings, birthdays or unique event suppers. A few people may encounter a "purging" response in the initial few days of cleanse, including headaches or loose bowel movements. This is because of the sudden withdrawal of specific nourishments, notwithstanding incitement of cleansing your organs. These indications inevitably die down in 24 to 48 hours.

THE CLEANSING TEA is not at all like another eating regimen arranges out there furnishes you with a small trick sheet to re-wiring your whole framework for fruitful weight reduction. Rather than starving yourself and subjecting your body to extreme changes in schedule, this gives a perfect structure to permit your body a move to return to such a framework, to the point that it begins performing better through and through and gives you the abundantly necessary change that you needed to find in your self-perception.

However, the advantages do not merely end here. The body reset arrangement enhances your resting, eating designs and for the most part just aides the body control itself. Undertaking this eating regimen arrangement may appear like very much an undertaking however at last as the idiom goes, the verification is in the pudding! Once you begin getting results, it will make you feel a great deal more sure about own self and the viability of this eating routine!

Final Words

Thank you again for purchasing this book! I really hope this book is able to help you.

The next step is for you to **join our email newsletter** to receive updates on any upcoming new book releases or promotions. You can sign-up for free and as a bonus, you will also receive our "*7 Fitness Mistakes You Don't Know You're Making*" book! This bonus book breaks down many of the most common fitness mistakes and will demystify many of the complexities and science of getting into shape. Having all this fitness knowledge and science organized into an actionable step-by-step book will help you get started in the right direction in your fitness journey! To join our free email newsletter and grab your free book, please visit the link and signup: **www.hmwpublishing.com/gift**

Finally, if you enjoyed this book, then I would like to ask you for a favor, would you be kind enough to leave a review for this book? It would be greatly appreciated!

Thank you and good luck in your journey!

About the Co-Author

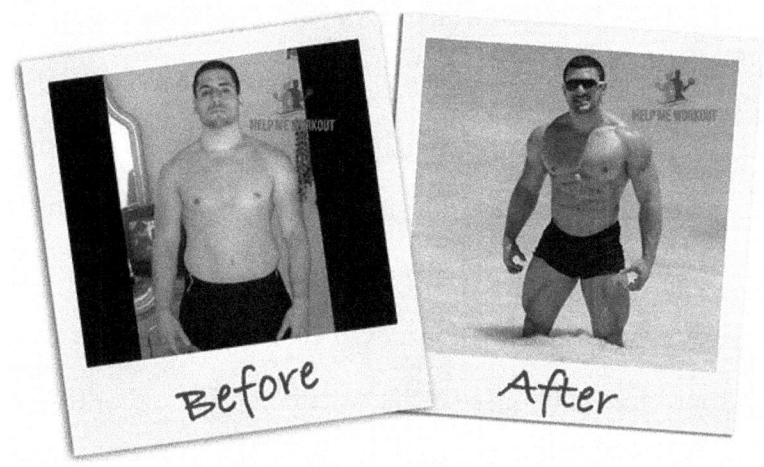

My name is George Kaplo; I'm a certified personal trainer from Montreal, Canada. I'll start off by saying I'm not the biggest guy you will ever meet and this has never really been my goal. In fact, I started working out to overcome my biggest insecurity when I was younger, which was my self-confidence. This was due to my height measuring only 5 foot 5 inches (168cm), it pushed me down to attempt anything I ever wanted to achieve in life. You may be going through some challenges right now, or you may simply want to get fit, and I can certainly relate.

For me personally, I was always kind of interested in the health & fitness world and wanted to gain some muscle due to the numerous bullying in my teenage years about my height and my overweight body. I figured I couldn't do anything about my height, but I sure can do something about how my body looked like. This was the beginning of my transformation journey. I had no idea where to start, but I just got started. I felt worried and afraid at times that other people would make fun of me for doing the exercises the wrong way. I always wished I had a friend that was next to me who was knowledgeable enough to help me get started and "show me the ropes."

After a lot of work, studying and countless trial and errors. Some people began to notice how I was getting more fit and how I was starting to form a keen interest in the topic. This led many friends and new faces to come to me and ask me for fitness advice. At first, it seemed odd when people asked me to help them get in shape. But what kept me going is when they started to see changes in their own body and told me it's the first time that they saw real results!

From there, more people kept coming to me, and it made me realize after so much reading and studying in this field that it did help me but it also allowed me to help others. I'm now a fully certified personal trainer and have trained numerous clients to date who have achieved amazing results.

Today, my brother Alex Kaplo (also a Certified Personal Trainer) and I own & operate this publishing venture, where we bring passionate and expert authors to write about health and fitness topics. We also run an online fitness website "HelpMeWorkout.com" and I would love to connect with by inviting you to visit the website on the following page and signing up to our e-mail newsletter (you will even get a free book).

Last but not least, if you are in the position I was once in and you want some guidance, don't hesitate and ask... I'll be there to help you out!

Your friend and coach,

George Kaplo
Certified Personal Trainer

Get another book for Free

I want to thank you for purchasing this book and offer you another book (just as long and valuable as this book), "Health & Fitness Mistakes You Don't Know You're Making", completely free.

Visit the link below to signup and receive it:

www.hmwpublishing.com/gift

In this book, I will break down the most common health & fitness mistakes, you are probably committing right now, and I will reveal how you can easily get in the best shape of your life!

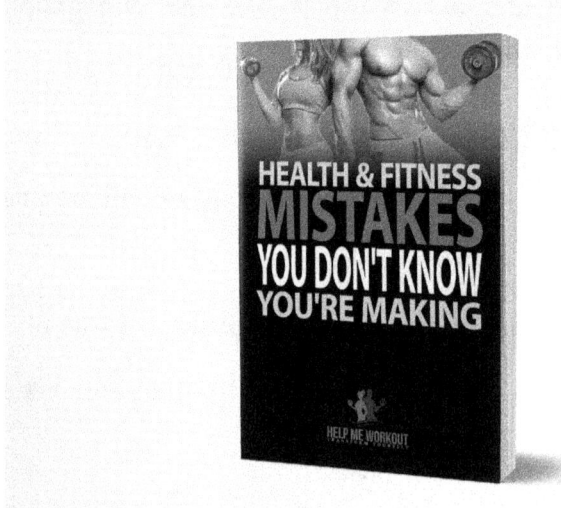

In addition to this valuable gift, you will also have an opportunity to get our new books for free, enter giveaways, and receive other valuable emails from me. Again, visit the link to sign up:

www.hmwpublishing.com/gift

Copyright 2017 by HMW Publishing - All Rights Reserved.

This document by HMW Publishing owned by the A&G Direct Inc company, is geared towards providing exact and reliable information in regards to the topic and issue covered. The publication is sold with the idea that the publisher is not required to render accounting, officially permitted, or otherwise, qualified services. If advice is necessary, legal or professional, a practiced individual in the profession should be ordered.

From a Declaration of Principles which was accepted and approved equally by a Committee of the American Bar Association and a Committee of Publishers and Associations.

In no way is it legal to reproduce, duplicate, or transmit any part of this document in either electronic means or in printed format. Recording of this publication is strictly prohibited, and any storage of this document is not allowed unless with written permission from the publisher. All rights reserved.

The information provided herein is stated to be truthful and consistent, in that any liability, in terms of inattention or otherwise, by any usage or abuse of any policies, processes, or directions contained within is the solitary and utter responsibility of the recipient reader. Under no circumstances will any legal responsibility or blame be held against the publisher for any reparation, damages, or monetary loss due to the information herein, either directly or indirectly.

The information herein is offered for informational purposes solely, and is universal as so. The presentation of the information is without contract or any type of guarantee assurance.

The trademarks that are used are without any consent, and the publication of the trademark is without permission or backing by the trademark owner. All trademarks and brands within this book are for clarifying purposes only and are the owned by the owners themselves, not affiliated with this document.

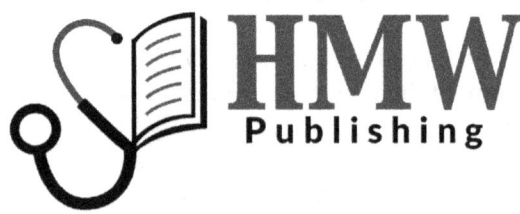

For more great books visit:

HMWPublishing.com

www.ingramcontent.com/pod-product-compliance
Lightning Source LLC
Chambersburg PA
CBHW071120030426
42336CB00013BA/2157